Edgar Cayce Cures

Cures

Using The Violet Ray
for Alternative Treatments

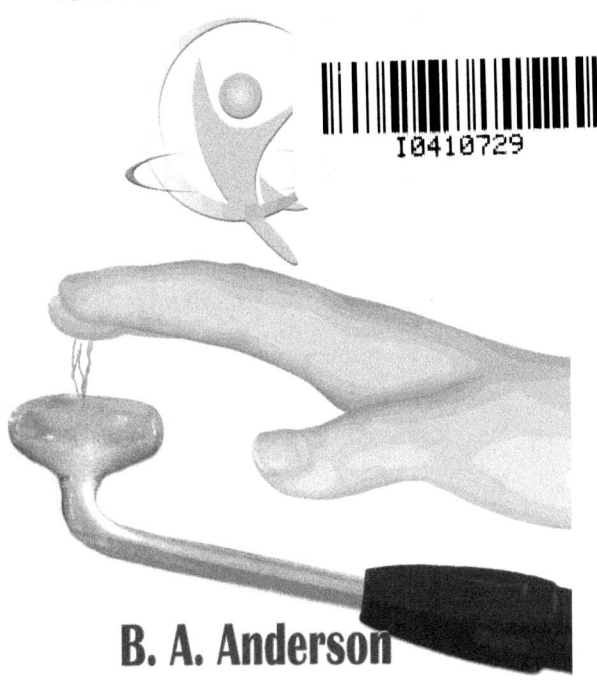

I0410729

B. A. Anderson

EdgarCayceCures.com

ISBN **978-1539301509** Paperback

Published by DM BookPro
Phoenix, AZ
DMBookPro.com

Available Now on Amazon Edgar

Cayce Cures - Using Alternative Holistic

Remedies and Treatments
Edgar Cayce Cures - All My Lives Journal
Using Akashic Records to Heal

Coming soon:

Edgar Cayce Cures - All My Lives Workbook
Edgar Cayce Cures - All My Lives Workshop CDs
Edgar Cayce Cures - Diabetes and Blood Sugar Levels
Edgar Cayce Cures – Using Ideals and Spiritual
Principles
Edgar Cayce Cures - Journal to Heal
Edgar Cayce Cures - Using Akashic Records

DEDICATION

This work and all of my work is dedicated to Spirit for all their Love, Guidance, and Protection and for that I am ever grateful! Thank you

INTRODUCTION

Body - Mind - Spirit

Spirit is the Life - Mind is the Builder - the Physical is the Result!

The Edgar Cayce Clinic (formally the A.R.E. Clinic) founded in 1970 by Drs. Bill and Gladys McGarey who treated it's patients for over 40 years following the readings of Edgar Cayce.

The Edgar Cayce Center of Arizona (A Holistic Educational Spiritual Center to continue the education of Edgar Cayce and his work) providing classes/events/discussions along with information on how to combine the Body - Mind - Spirit practices associated with Edgar Cayce's work. You may find more information about the Center:

EdgarCayceCures.com or **EdgarCayceCenter.com** or **Meetup.com/EdgarCayceCenter**

The Readings: Available for examination and study at the Association for Research and Enlightenment, Inc.,(A.R.E.®) at Virginia Beach, Va. There are 14,256 readings consisting of 49,135 pages of verbatim psychic material plus related correspondence.

The Violet Ray is available for purchase at www.edgarcaycecures.com just click on the Cayce Store drop down.

CONTENTS

DISCLAIMER

Although the Violet Ray was recommended in over 900 readings by Edgar Cayce, (the Father of Holistic medicine) and The Edgar Cayce Clinic successfully used the Violet Ray for over Forty years in their holistic practice of treating patients. The FDA has only approved the Violet Ray device for limited use. The Violet Ray is approved as a device for dermatological therapy such as removal of warts, moles, blemishes and fungus of the skin. It is also approved for hair regrowth or hair stimulation.

Further as a precaution, there are some conditions or concerns you must consider before using the Violet Ray.

They are:
The Violet Ray may cause tingling or sparking around any metal if have any metal plates or pins.

The Violet Ray should not make direct contact with any metal, so do not use near any metal jewelry.

The Violet Ray has a high-frequency and cannot be used if you have a pacemaker or have an electronic hearing implant.

The Violet Ray should not be used if you have drunk any alcohol. Fatal complications can occur if alcohol is in your blood.

There could be a risk to pregnant women if they use the Violet Ray.

If you have a heart murmur or heart disease, the Violet Ray should be used from the back only. Do not move the Violet Ray directly over the heart.

EDGAR CAYCE

The medical intuitive Edgar Cayce provided more than 9000 health readings claiming that Body - Mind - Spirit are equally important to healing. Cayce developed concepts and a healing approach that applies to physical, emotional and spiritual problems.

When Cayce was a teenager he had a vision of an Angel that said his prayers had been answered. She asked what his prayer might be and offered to help him. Edgar told the Angel that he wanted to help people, heal the sick, especially children.

Several years later while he was hypnotized to find the cause of losing his voice, his psychic gift appeared. In a hypnotic state Edgar Cayce diagnosed and recommended a post-hypnotic suggestion that returned his voice to normal. Cayce had just given his first health reading and thought perhaps he could do the same for others by going into a trance state, scanning the body and having the recommendation to help that person.

Then for each reading he performed, he would loosen his belt, collar, remove his cufflinks and untie his shoelaces. Then he would lie down on the couch and fold his hands over his stomach. Cayce would still his mind, close his eyes and give himself the suggestion to begin the reading.

Much of what Cayce talked about that related to diet, exercise and meditation are an important part of our modern holistic program. Cayce thought that Body-Mind-Spirit were crucial to any health condition. Additionally, Edgar's ideas on electrical therapies and energy medicine proved to be a beneficial aid to holistically heal.

Great results have been experienced from the interplay of Body-Mind-Spirit medicine from the Cayce readings. Edgar would say that Spirit is the Life, Mind is the Builder and the Physical is the Result and this would summarize Cayce's viewpoint.

Cayce implied that the words we speak and our state of mind reflect a deeper level of a cause than the foods that are eaten. This does not mean that a proper diet is not crucial to a healthy body, but as important as the spiritual and mental factors.

There is no such thing as only physical or only mental disease, because all physical ailments have mental parts, just as mental ailments have physical aspects. Cayce's holistic approach looks at the mental and physical attributes of an illness to cure it.

Between 1901 and 1944 more than 14,000 readings were transcribed and given to over six thousand seekers. Each reading had a number assigned based on the person who it was given to and the number of readings that person had. Such as 1011-3 would relate to the one thousand and eleventh person to get a reading and the three would signify his third reading, this would be done to protect the identity of the person receiving the reading. The readings cover a broad range of topics mostly health related and another large group called life readings related to previous incarnations that would indicate how previous lifetimes would affect present lifetimes, known as Akashic record readings. Dream interpretation, business advice, and spiritual advice were the other reading types.

Edgar Cayce, called the "Sleeping Prophet", for close to 43 years he was able to read the body of the person requesting his help. He would then suggest remedies or treatments and changes in diet that related to the condition in question.

Those of who wish to learn more about Edgar Cayce Health, treatments and remedies visit www.edgarcaycecures.com.

THE VIOLET RAY

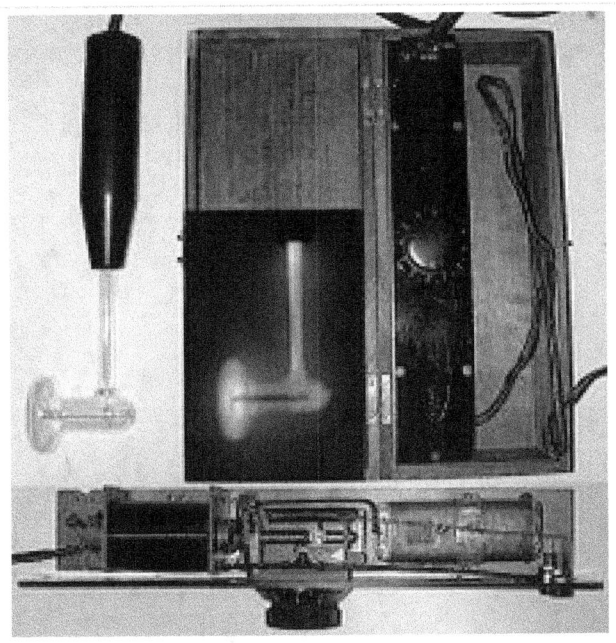

A Violet Ray is an electrotherapy medical appliance used during the early 20th century. Nikola Tesla invented the basic construction of the Violet Ray prior to 1900. Tesla's coil is really an electrical **resonant transformer** circuit. Using a disruptive discharge coil with an **interrupter** that applies a low current, a high voltage, with a high frequency.

Tesla introduced the first prototypes at the **World's Columbian Exposition** in 1893. During the Depression-era the first Violet Rays were produced in the US.

Using an ungrounded wooden electrical box that could control the interrupter and that which housed the magneto coil, and an attached plastic handle/housing which contained the high voltage coil and an insertion port for various attachments. Varying shapes of glass evacuated tubes could be used for different therapeutic uses by inserting them into the plastic handle.

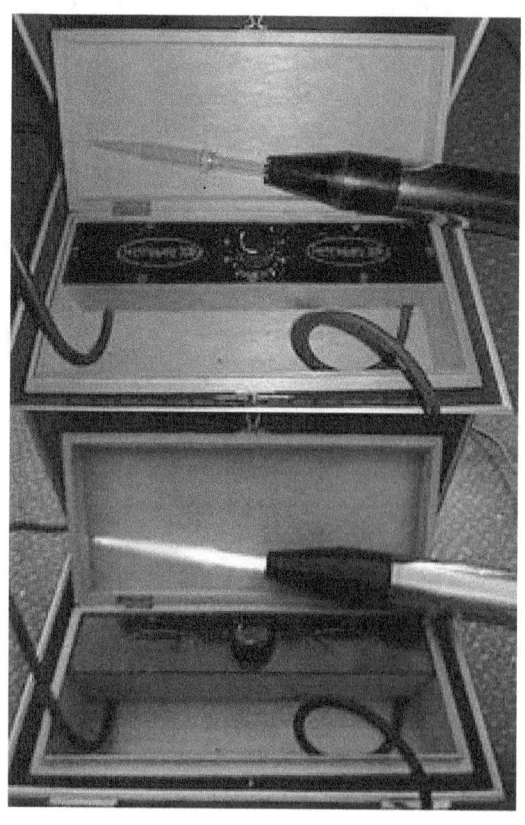

The Violet Ray is just one of the several electrical appliances recommended in the over 9000 **Edgar Cayce** health related readings. The **Edgar Cayce Clinic** also used the Violet Ray during its electrotherapy sessions on its patients for pain, skin conditions and spinal issues. With the rather unique varied shaped electrodes this unique instrument; was used during **Cayce's** day by physicians and laypeople from pharmacies or electrical appliance stores. Cosmetologists use it today for acne, wrinkles, psoriasis, and stimulating hair growth and rejuvenation.

THE VIOLET RAY APPLIANCE

The Violet Ray appliance is a high-frequency, high voltage, the low current source of static electricity. It can be applied to any part of the body. The name Violet Ray comes from the violet color of the electrical discharge that is emitted during its use. The Violet Ray device was recommended by Edgar Cayce in over 900 Psychic readings for a wide variety of problems that might require stimulation to the circulatory and nervous systems.

The importance of using the violet ray treatment is that it brings a vigorous surge of rich, warm blood to any part of the body. Thereby it washes away the sediment of a disease, then strengthens and nourishes the tissues, and gives vigor and vitality to any part of the body that is treated.

The Violet Ray device consists of a cylindrical base which is held in your hand. Various shaped glass tubes can be inserted into the end of the plastic unit that has an opening for the tube. Originally, a diversity of the glass tubes were used for various treatments, various sizes, and shaped electrodes can be used for almost every portion of the body. Currently, the electrotherapy device comes with a set of simple bulb vacuum tubes in various shapes.

Violet Ray Accomplishments

Violet Rays benefit all living matter and through the glass vacuum applicator, the light, heat, electric energy and ozone are created. The Violet Ray give us a remedy that we can rely on. They will reach where medicine cannot and yet cause no pain or discomfort while destroying infection with soothing relief.

The vibration of the Violet Ray will cause the millions of cells in the body to vibrate and its frequency is so high that we are unaware that the effect is rapid and powerful.

Violet Ray Effects

With daily treatments you can expect:

- ❖ return of regular sleep pattern
- ❖ strength and vital energy increasing
- ❖ cheerfulness and work attitude will increase
- ❖ appetite and digestion improvement
- ❖ blood supply improvement
- ❖ the nervous system becomes more soothed
- ❖ oxygen in the blood increases
- ❖ wrinkles and puffiness in the face are reduced
- ❖ helps to relieve swelling, pain and inflammation by promoting circulation
- ❖ will tighten facial muscles, including the muscles under the chin.
- ❖ stimulates circulation to the scalp and promotes hair growth.
- ❖ generate a sense of well-being and reduce stress

THE ELECTRODES

The Small Mushroom

The Large Mushroom

The Comb/Rake

The Ear or Curve

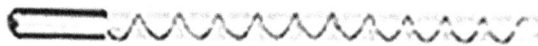

The Internal or Straight

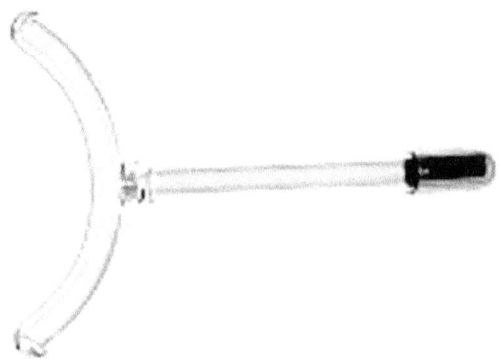

The Y or Throat or Curve

The Roller

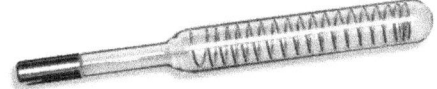

The Yoni or Prostrate

HOW TO CARE FOR THE GLASS ELECTRODES

Cleaning the Violet Ray electrodes is very important especially if the Violet Ray instrument is used by more than one person.

All the glass electrodes can be boiled in water to sterilize them, and to keep from spreading any infection.

Rinse the electrodes in warm water and soap, drying with a towel will guard against most troubles. In cases of skin and scalp diseases, you should use Lysol. The best way would be to place in a silverware rack in a dishwasher, so as not to touch each other to keep from breaking. They should also go through the drying heat drying cycle to further sterilize.

VIOLET RAY TREATMENTS
QUICK TREATMENT CHART
Using the mushroom electrode

Complexion: Use the mushroom electrode and apply to face and neck.

Headache: Use mushroom electrode and apply to 8, 5, 13, 12, 11, 20 for 2 to 3 minutes.

Hair, Dandruff, and Scalp: The mushroom electrode can be used, but the rake/comb electrode can cover the area better and treat the hair also. Treatment should last about eight minutes over entire scalp at least once a day.

Insomnia: Use the electrode and apply to 18, 19 and 7, 8. Move the electrode from 11, 10, 9, 6 and 4 to relieve insomnia.

Indigestion: Use the mushroom electrode and apply to area 18, 19 and 20 for 5 minutes. Then also apply along the spine 4, 6, 9, 10, and 11 to further treat indigestion.

Nervousness: Treatment should begin on area 12 for about 5 minutes, then continue using the mushroom electrode on 11, 10 then up and down the spine 10, 9, 6, and 4. The outer areas of the back 7, 8, 13 and also 29, 30 this completes the back area for 2 to 3 minutes per area. Apply also to the front abdominal areas by laying the mushroom electrode to 16, 17 18, and 19. Treating the upper arm areas 24 and 25 can also help the nervousness along with treating the lower limbs area 1 and 2.

Rheumatism: Apply a thin layer of cloth to the area to treat pain by applying the mushroom electrode to 18,19, 7 and 8.

Face Neuralgia: Apply to sides of the neck, both cheeks and in front of both ears.

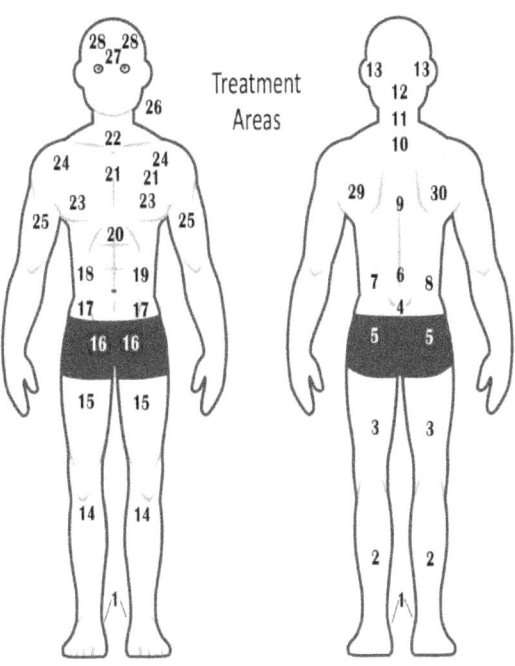

Treatment Areas

DIRECTIONS

1. Holding the handle of the appliance insert the Glass Applicator into the handle of the machine.

2. Insert the plug into an 110 electrical outlet.

3. Turn the knob at the bottom of the unit to turn it on.

4. By turning this knob you will increase the intensity of the Violet Ray strength.

5. If you use hair tonic that contains alcohol, you must not use the Violet Ray.

6. Start with a lower setting or mild current to begin all treatments and then increase to desired strength. Follow instructions for each specific treatment in the next section.

7. If you hold the electrode away from your skin or body there may be an arc or spark when it connects to the skin.

8. If you hold the electrode right next to the skin, you will receive a much deeper treatment rather than topical.

9. When the treatment is done, turn off the switch on the bottom of the unit, and then unplug from the outlet.

10. **ALWAYS** insert the electrode with a straight push into the handle and then use a straight pull to remove the electrode. YOU SHOULD NEVER TWIST the electrode.

11. To avoid shock, remove metallic objects such rings, watches, jewelry, hairpins, chains.

SKIN TREATMENTS

Abscesses

Use the mushroom electrode and contact the skin. Gently move over the electrode over the entire affected area for 3 - 5 minutes. The current must be very mild. When applied to a developing abscess, its growth can be arrested. This electrode also comes in a larger size.

Acne (Pimples)

Treat the entire skin surface for about 6 minutes with the mushroom electrode. Raise the electrode slightly to give a small spark for a short time, where pustules are forming. You should use a thin towel or handkerchief over the pustules. This effect will soon cause the pimples to ripen and disappear. When you do the treatment through a towel or handkerchief it seems disagreeable, apply the mushroom applicator directly on the skin but first, powder the skin with talcum powder. This creates a dryer surface and prevents the sticking of the applicator to damp skin.

Anaemia

To increase the oxygenation of the blood, treat with the mushroom electrode for 4 - 6 minutes. Applications made to the naked surface of the body should be dried and you should use talcum powder. The Violet Ray's regenerative forces help produce new blood cells.

Barber's Itch

Providing treatment through a handkerchief or a piece of cotton is advisable. You cannot remove it in one treatment. Apply treatment to the affected area daily using the mushroom electrode for about 5 minutes. Creating the small sparks over the whole surface and especially towards the edges are very helpful.

Birth Marks

Using a medium current and the mushroom electrode repeated at convenience and often.

Blackheads

A mild to a medium current applied using the mushroom electrode for 3 - 5 minutes. Use it once a day. to remove blackheads. You can use castor oil over the areas before you treat them.

Bunions

Move the applicator slowly over the painful area while keeping in contact with the skin. Using the mushroom electrode with a medium current for about 6 minutes will relieve all pain.

Bruises

A gentle back and forth movement while touching the skin is sufficient. Use the mushroom electrode with mild or medium current applied to bring immediate results to the painful swollen spots.

Burns

A gentle current for a short time period, about 2 to 3 minutes 2 or 3 times a day and applied using the mushroom electrode does a lot of good and tends to relieve the pain. Apply Castor Oil for added healing relief.

Callouses

Using a strong current with the mushroom electrode on its edge to spark the skin directly for 1 or 2 minutes. Repeat as necessity requires.

Corns

Turn the mushroom electrode on its edge so that the spark emits from its edge instead of coming from its face. Hold it about 1/8 inch from the corn to allow short sparks to emit for a few seconds only into the corn. Repeat this in a day or two with close contact for 2 to 3 minutes to relieve pain.

Eczema

To start lay a piece of thin cloth over the affected area and treat with the mushroom shaped electrode. Use a mild current at first, then increase the current strength if it can be tolerated. If the skin itches you can bring quick relief by lifting the electrode slightly from the cloth. In nearly all cases to effect a cure, treat the area daily for 3 to 5 minutes.

Freckles

Cover the skin surface with gauze. Use the mushroom electrode daily from 4 - 6 minutes with a medium current. Results are slow to come.

Frost Bites

Use the mushroom shaped electrode with a medium current strength, allowing short sparks to pass to the frost affected parts for 3 to 5 minutes, every two or three hours to bring lasting results in a very short time.

Furunculosis

For Boils, treat with the mushroom electrode. Mild or medium current strength. The inflammation will cease quickly.

Hives and Rash

Use the mushroom electrode with a medium current strength to affected area. Use Castor Oil before applying the treatment for 3 - 5 minutes should be sufficient. Repeat every day.

Red Nose (Acne Rosacea)

Use the mushroom electrode and apply for only short periods, say about 2 minutes at a time. By holding the mushroom electrode sideways and hold away from skin about an eighth of an inch, you can obtain small sparks. The object is to destroy the enlarged veins. The treatment must not be performed for a long length of time. It should be repeated as the condition permits. It is advisable to rest for several days between treatments.

Poison Ivy

Apply a bit of castor oil first, then you can cause sparking by turning the mushroom electrode on its edge. Continue the sparking over the entire affected area. By lifting the electrode here and there to treat for 3 - 5 minutes, this changes the current strength. Relief is immediate and always a pleasure.

Ringworm

Use the mushroom electrode and medium current, lift the electrode from the skin so you can make short sparks for several minutes. The treatment should repeat every other day, three to four times a day, make sure to cover all the affected areas.

Skin Disease

Using the mushroom electrode for most skin disease types, the high-Frequency spray or (small sparks) is most successful the sparking action promotes skin tissue connectivity. You should pass the electrode rapidly back and forth over the affected area for several minutes. Use talcum powder if the skin is moist so that the electrode will not stick. Another method is to spread gauze over the skin area to be treated. This will allow the electrode to smoothly glide and at the same time does not remove the electrode away from skin enough to cause the spark.

In the case of itching lift the electrode away from skin enough to cause longer and sharper sparks. Apply for shorter periods of time. Use this same method to Epithelioma, Lupus and Chronic Ulcers.

Warts

Use the mushroom electrode and hold it about one-eighth of an inch away from the warts and allow sparks to pass from the edge of the glass. For the best results use the smaller tipped spoon or ear electrode. Let the point rest directly on top of the wart and use a weak current. But use a stronger current through any deeper crustation. Just a few seconds are usually sufficient. You can repeat after 2 or 3 days.

Wrinkles

Are commonly caused by using any given set of facial muscles more often than normal. They can be treated by applying the mushroom electrode right over them with a circular, massaging motion. The high-frequency current revitalizes tired muscles and arrests the blighted marks of time.

Hair Treatments

Alopecia (Falling Hair)

Use the comb/rake electrode with a weak current at first , and increase to a medium strength later. Move the comb back and forth over the entire scalp for about 4 or 5 minutes every day. You can use the same treatment for baldness and for gray hair in order to restore the hair to its natural color. If you have used hair tonic you should NOT use the Violet Ray.

Dandruff

Before the treatment, you should shampoo the hair and scalp, dry your hair thoroughly and then by using the comb/rake applicator apply a medium current. Then comb your hair using the comb/rake electrode for 3 to 5 minutes. Be sure not to use any hair tonic. Treatment should be repeated every 2 - 3 days.

Gray Hair

Use a current of sufficient strength for good stimulation every day once or twice a day. It is possible to restore the natural color of hair using the comb/rake electrode. It may take 2 months before you see results. Make sure scalp is kept clean.

Scalp Treatment

Dandruff, falling hair, gray hair, baldness, itching scalp, etc., gain great benefits from the Violet Rays. There is no question that the Violet Ray represents the most scientific method of treating the scalp. Its beneficial value is beyond all doubt. Violet Rays produce a normal and healthy scalp, and revitalize impoverished hair, to restore its natural luster and fullness. This stimulates new hair growth by allowing new nutrients to flow to the dormant papilla cells.

Using the comb/rake electrode every day one to three times a day for several minutes. Do not use any hair tonic. Violet Rays constitute the best hair tonic all by themselves.

In the case of baldness, the Violet Ray proves to be very effective in the regrowth of hair. Continued use of Violet Ray high-frequency current and patience have surprised many users.

Gray hair has returned to its original color and beauty in many cases. We do not claim too much by saying that routine scalp applications with the comb/rake electrode are the only reliable means to stimulate and assist the natural growth of hair at the present time.

PAIN

Backache

To treat sore muscles in the back through bath towel with either the small or larger mushroom electrode and cover the entire area that is in pain. This will relieve the pain. As backaches may have different causes, such as weakness of the bladder or lumbago, rheumatism, kidney disease, it is of important to treat these causes also.

Gout

Apply to the painful area using the mushroom electrode with a medium current keeping the applicator in contact but moving it slowly about. The pain may increase slightly at first but you should feel relief after just a few treatments.

Headaches

There are varying causes for headaches. If relief is not felt by applying the mushroom electrode to the seat of a headache, using a medium current for 5 - 7 minutes.

Lumbago

To relieve the pain, use the larger mushroom electrode until all the pain is dispelled. Repeat treatment whenever pain appears until cured.

Neuralgia

Apply to the seat of pain, raising the mushroom electrode occasionally to produce a spark on the painful area.

Neuritis

The first few treatments you may not feel relief but an increase in pain. Once relief is felt the current may be increased and a short spark given on applied areas. Using the small or larger mushroom electrode apply at the seat of pain.

Pains

Using either mushroom electrode, the high-frequency current is wonderful to relieve pain. Apply the mushroom electrode to the area of pain until relief is felt. Apply electrode directly to the skin for best relief. Medium current strength and sometimes strong currents are advised.

Rheumatism

A strong current has to be used in all cases of Rheumatism. This disease responds quickly, especially the muscular and chronic articular form. In acute cases of this ailment, the results are slower to obtain but nevertheless satisfactory. The affected body parts or areas should be treated until all the pain ceases. Changing the position of body parts or extremities being treated will likely expose other body parts or areas requiring treatment. Stretching the muscles and using the high-frequency current long enough to relieve all the discomfort. The larger mushroom applicator is especially recommended for these treatments. You can repeat these applications as often as pain reappears. Only use the instrument for 10 minutes at one time. The applicator can be used directly on the skin but some cases may require using the applicator through clothing or several layers of a towel.

Sciatica

This term sometimes describes the symptom of any pain in the low back that continues down the leg. Other times the term describes a nerve dysfunction, compression of lumbar. The sciatic nerves begin at the low back run down the outside of the thigh from hip to the front of the knee. They lie near the bones and deep under the heavy muscles. The slightest pressure on the sciatic nerves can cause extreme pain, they become inflamed and tender. Using the small or larger mushroom electrode applied through the clothing or over the painful area will bring quick relief.

Stiff Neck, Joints

Apply in the same manner as under "Neuritis," using the mushroom electrode. Use a longer treatment, if necessary. In cases of a stiff neck rub the small mushroom electrode along the back of the ear and down the neck on both sides for 3 to 5 minutes with a strong current.

Sore Feet and Bruises

Apply with any sized electrode, suitable for the area. Keep the applicator in close contact with the skin to bring quick relief. Use Castor Oil as a lubricant and treat for several minutes.

Sprains

Close contact applications with a mushroom applicator prove helpful, allowing deep penetration. Use a medium current and in some cases lift the electrode to cause small sparks during treatment through a towel for 4 or 5 minutes usually, suffices.

CHEST

Asthma

Use the mushroom electrode over the chest and the throat electrode on the throat glands for about 6 minutes. Use a strong current if it can be tolerated. If treatment is taken when the attack is near, much relief can be had and sometimes the attack can be entirely averted.

Bronchitis

Create short sparks with the large mushroom electrode applied through a Turkish towel over the chest and back, sufficient to produce a reddening of the skin.

Colds in Lungs

Treat the chest and back using the mushroom electrode using a strong current for 5 to 6 minutes.

Consumption

The patient receiving treatment must be naked to the waist line. The skin should be dried and powdered with talcum powder all over. Using the large mushroom electrode, apply the high frequency current to the chest.

Start with medium current strength and increase to a stronger current to aid in the discharge of phlegm. This will activate the secretion glands into action and it will improve the nutrient blood supply through the tissues. Move the applicator around the chest and the flow towards the throat. Breathe deeply to fill the lungs as much as possible. Move from chest towards both sides of the body and also the gastric region repeatedly. Then after 5 - 6 minutes of using the applicator over the front of the body. The patient should turn over and continue the application on the back of the body. A strong current should be used along the spinal nerve centers from top to the base, also over the shoulder blades, and include the low back, over the kidney area.

Pleurisy

Use the large mushroom electrode and cover the back and the chest with a Turkish towel. Then use a vigorous treatment through the Turkish towel until the skin becomes quite red. Treat for 8 to 10 minutes and keep the electrode moving.

Pneumonia

Apply the very same treatment as given under Pleurisy. When using a high-frequency current you can expect to do wonders, even with grave diseases.

Tuberculosis(See Consumption.)

Whooping Cough

Apply the small mushroom electrode in the same way as explained under "Asthma"

THROAT

Mumps

Treat swollen parts using the small mushroom electrode for 2 to 3 minutes.

Tonsillitis

Use the throat electrode and move it up and down the throat area for about 5 minutes.

Sore Throat

The throat electrode is best suited for all external throat applications. Castor Oil can be used as a lubricant and the throat electrode is moved up and down the throat in close contact, for 5 or 6 minutes. Be sure to cover all of the throat areas with a medium or strong current: repeat 2 or 3 times a day.

STOMACH

Ulcers

Apply a strong current with the large mushroom electrode for 5 minutes in contact. Make sure to lift the applicator once in a while to produce sparks, and you can repeat this treatment every day.

MOUTH

Pyorrhea

Use the ear electrode inside the mouth and allow sparks to gums. A weak or medium current can help greatly to re-establish a healthy condition of the gums

OTHER

Arteriosclerosis (High Blood Pressure or Hardening of the Arteries)

Apply the mushroom electrode over the body generally, using a medium current strength. Daily treatments of about 5 minutes' duration will serve to lower the blood pressure.

Ataxia

Use as strong a current as it can be tolerated for this treatment. Apply using the mushroom electrode over both sides of the entire spine. Daily treatments should last about 10 minutes for the first few days. The time can gradually decrease with progressing improvement.

Bladder Disease (Cystitis)

Treat using the small or large mushroom electrode with a strong current all over the area of the bladder for 5 minutes twice a day. Relief is usually quick with a strong current and the urine will clear fast .

Brain Fog

Use a medium current and the mushroom applicator over the forehead and eyes. Continue application to the back of the head, down the neck and also down the spine for about 8 to 10 minutes.

Breast Development

You should use the large mushroom electrode and move the electrode to cover the entire breast area to be developed for about 5 - 7 minutes daily. Starting from the neck downward move it lightly from side to side. Be sure to include from arm pit to arm pit, and under each breast, pressing lightly upward towards the nipple.

Canker

Use a small electrode like the ear electrode with a medium current for one or two minutes.

Cataract

For surprising results close the eyelids and use a small electrode with a weak current for 3 to 4 minutes.

Cold Extremities

Use the large mushroom electrode and a strong current for about 5 minutes over the entire part of the body affected. You should produce a reddening of the skin, by keeping the applicator in contact with the skin while moving the electrode. Repeat, 3 times a day if necessary.

Colds in Head

Use a medium current 2 or 3 times a day over the nose, above eyes and the sides of the face. Use either the small or large mushroom electrode.

Deafness

Using the Ear electrode with a mild current gives excellent results. Use for about 3 minutes, and insert the electrode deep into the ear. If the heating effect becomes too much to handle, stop the treatment and repeat again later. Treatments at least twice daily should be sufficient. You can also use the small mushroom electrode on the back of the ear.

Earache or Ear Diseases

Insert the ear electrode and a mild current for short periods of time. Use the small mushroom electrode to the back of the ear will benefit the ear pain.

Eye Diseases

The Violet Ray has successfully been used to treat Iritis, Retinitis, Atrophy of the Optic Nerve. Conjunctivitis, Trachoma, Glaucoma, Incipient Cataract, You should close your eyelids and apply a mild current and use the spoon electrode 2 to 3 minutes. Do not exceed 3 minutes at one time. You can repeat as desirable.

Goitre

For about 4 minutes at a time, use the throat electrode with a strong current. It may be more comfortable to lay gauze on the throat and then apply treatment with the strongest current. By the 10th or 12th treatment, the results should be noticeable.

Grippe (Influenza)

Treatment to the spine and solar plexus by using the mushroom electrode. Also, treat over the eyelids and down the sides of the nose. Use a Turkish towel over the spine and solar plexus area for 5 -7 minutes two or more times a day. For 1 to 2 minutes with a weak current and the ear electrode intra nasally.

Hay Fever

Apply the mushroom electrode over the nose and along the spine with medium current for 5 minutes and use the ear electrode in nostrils for a short period of time. Applications should be of short duration but repeated often. It is advisable to anticipate the season and to begin treatments before attacks are expected or any discomfort felt.

Infantile Paralysis

Weak and feeble muscles can regain strength by using the high frequency applicator with the mushroom electrode for 5 to 7 minutes. Place directly over entire area to be worked on.

Inflammations

Can be reduced and relieved by application with the mushroom electrode. Move the electrode slowly over the inflamed area, keep it in close contact and use a medium current for 5 to 6 minutes.

Insomnia

Cover the back of the head, neck, and eyebrows by using the mushroom electrode with a strong current. Treatment should be 5 - 7 minutes for best results.

Impotence

A beneficial way to treat Impotence is to use the Insert electrode. Use the mushroom electrode, slightly raised and with plenty of sparks. Move the electrode over the area of the genital and the spine for 5 - 7 minutes daily.

Massage

Turn on the current using the mushroom electrode and glide over the area to be massaged. The area will be stimulated and warmed to deepen the massage effect.

Nervousness

Treat the spine, back of head and neck area using the mushroom electrode for 5 to 7 minutes. Immediate results will be felt by the stimulation.

Obesity

Apply the mushroom electrode to the affected parts and treat consistently. Begin as indicated and increase current as strong as you can tolerate. The fatty tissue will decrease and redistribute, giving you greater comfort.

Paralysis

Using the mushroom electrode along the affected muscles. A strong current is necessary. Keep the electrode moving. Treat area for about 6 minutes, use Castor Oil and apply to the affected part so that the electrode slides easily. Obtaining sparks through a Turkish towel will help quickly. Use this method every day.

RECTAL

Constipation

Use the large mushroom attachment and apply a strong current over the entire abdominal area. Treatment should be for least 6 minutes, keeping the electrode moving at all times.

Physicians can use the rectal electrode well lubricated before insertion into the rectum for 5 minutes the treatment is sufficient.

Fistulas

Physicians can use the rectal electrode that is well lubricated before insertion into the rectum. Use a medium current for about 5 minutes daily.

Piles (Hemorrhoids and other rectal diseases)

Physicians can use the rectal electrode well lubricated before insertion into the rectum for 5 minutes the treatment is sufficient.

TESTIMONIALS

I used to walk with a cane because I had arthritis in my left knee. I visited a friend who owned a violet ray and they offered to do a treatment on my knee. After only 10 minutes of using the violet ray, I have no pain in my knee. I don't need a cane anymore and I seem to have more energy.

Roger Lee

My neighbor lady was suffering from low back pain and suffered from moving. My wife used the Violet Ray on her low back and in about ten minutes she was able to move pain-free. My neighbor was so relieved. She recommends The Violet Ray because it worked like a charm.

Charles Woodell

Pain Relief

I had been living with pain for many years. I recently discovered the Violet Ray and tried it on my low back and knees. I find it to provide soothing pain relief. I feel better than I have for years. Using the Violet Ray for last three weeks and I am feeling so much better.

S. Toran

Cures Neuritis; Relieved Throat

I wish to advise you that after using one of the Violet Ray machines for a short time that I am completely cured of Neuritis. It has also assisted wonderfully in relieving my throat before singing.

Varicose Veins

I have had some experience with a Violet Ray machine as a treatment for Varicose Veins and worked wonderfully.

In less than one minute this lady was remarking how good she was feeling and in twenty minutes looked as if nothing had happened, in fact, said she felt better than she had for some time. I believe it would be a favor to inform the public of this experience and should convince any skeptical persons as to the merits of this machine.

To see more recent testimonials, please go to

edgarcaycecures.com/violet-ray

NICOLA TESLA

Born on July 10, 1856, Nikola Tesla in Smiljan, Lika, which was then part of the Austo-Hungarian Empire, region of Croatia.

A visionary and a brilliant inventor, Tesla is known as the father of scalar, zero-point technology, and the Tesla Coil. The Violet Ray uses the technology of static electricity as the source that is high frequency and low amperage. Edgar Cayce (1877-1945) a peer of Tesla, recommended the use of the violet ray in almost 900 of his 14,000 readings. The original violet ray devices were indicated and suggested in many Cayce readings.

Tesla's guess was that he could pass his high frequency current into the body harmlessly and that they could be used for therapeutic healing.

Tesla decided to experiment on himself, after being struck down by a taxi near his hotel room. He did not go to a hospital, instead, in seclusion, he began to work on himself. After dragging himself to his hotel room he recovered from the contusions and fractures by using his electrotherapy device.

He never patented in electrotherapy but in 1891 began publishing his observations in technical journals, and seven years later we find Tesla giving a speech to the American Electrotherapeutic Association in which he details with drawings the high-frequency apparatus he has invented for this purpose, which included a Tesla coil.

Nikola Tesla met with Paul Oudin after realizing that the high-frequency electricity had amazing effects on health. They met in Paris in 1892 to discuss building high-frequency therapeutic oscillators. A few months later the Violet Ray was created by Oudin.

Experiments began with skin disorders such as acne, eczema, and even psoriasis, the new device could treat these easily. When the device was used on skin cancer or warts and allowed to spark after about three weeks of use they were removed. In two to three months skin patches would break up or disappear.

Oudin's device using the Tesla high-frequency electricity would also relieve pain and was considered a miracle device.

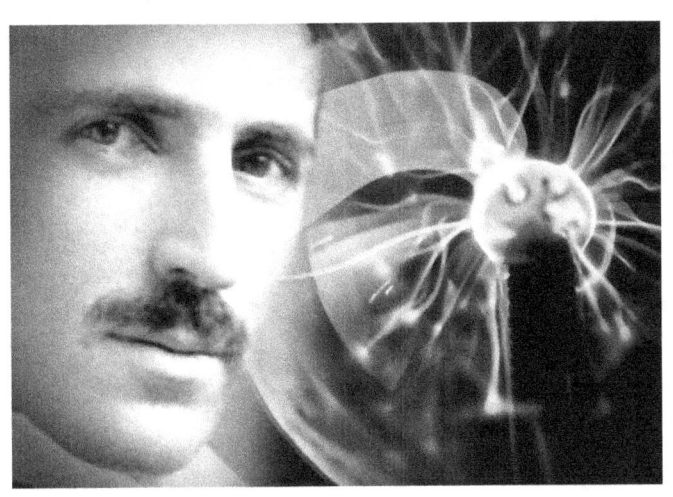

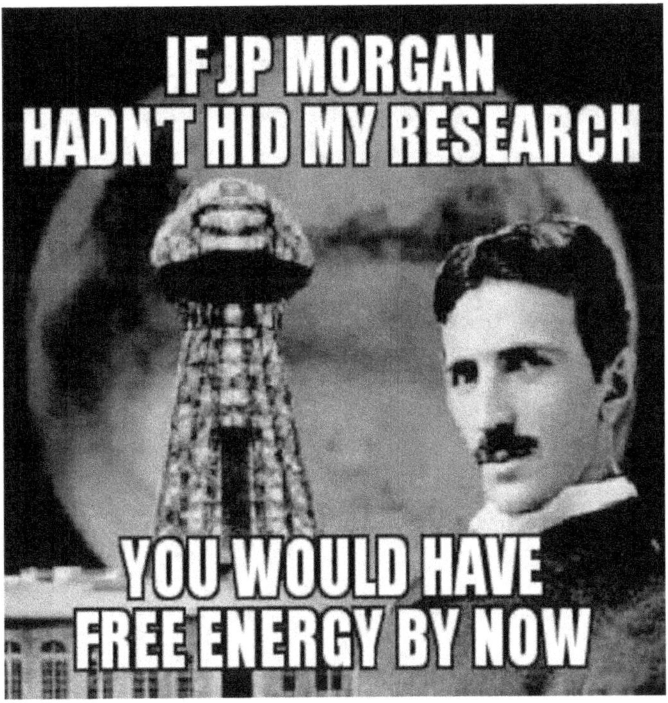

IF JP MORGAN
HADN'T HID MY RESEARCH

YOU WOULD HAVE
FREE ENERGY BY NOW

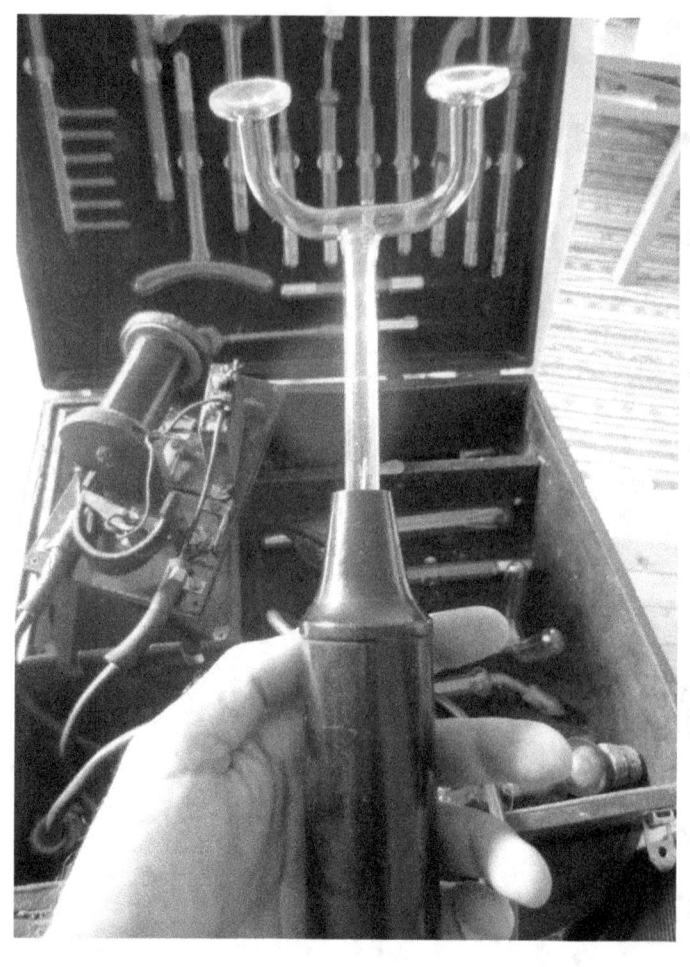

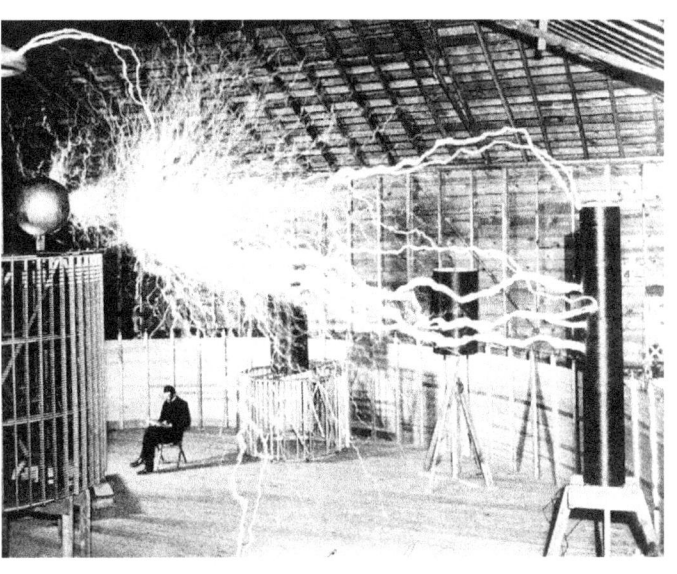

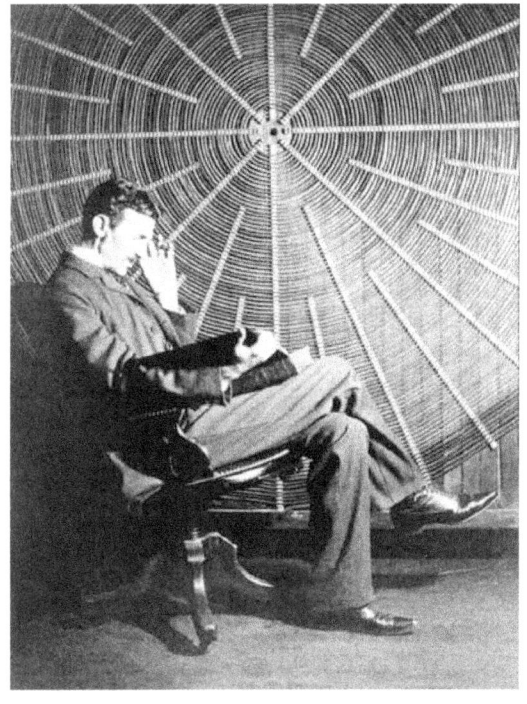

EDGAR CAYCE CENTER

The Temple Beautiful Program ®

The residential Temple Beautiful Program was developed by Dr. William McGarey of the Edgar Cayce Clinic who described it as an eleven-day "rejuvenation program" that includes dream analysis, akashic record work, stress reduction, visualization, meditation, biofeedback, exercise, diet, sound therapy, crystal work, nutrition, and supplementation. The program had been conducted more than two hundred times over the past decade, and it accommodates ten to fifteen participants in a group setting.

This program will be implemented to serve in as an online study program and also an in person retreat program. Look for more information on this program and other Edgar Cayce based workshops, classes and materials at **EdgarCayceCenter.com**